I0704263

DASH Diet: The Complete Beginners Guide to Dash Dieting, including Meal Plan and Recipes for Weight Loss and Clean Eating

Contents

Introduction

Thank you for choosing and welcome to **DASH Diet: The Complete Beginners Guide to Dash Dieting, including Meal Plan and Recipes for Weight Loss and Clean Eating**. Let's get straight to it!

The standard western diet is absolutely packed with processed ingredients that lead to and exacerbate hypertension and other related health problems. Hypertension (HTN, HT) otherwise known as high blood pressure is a problem that affects over 1 billion people worldwide; a number which increases every year. This is a serious concern the world over as those who suffer from Hypertension are at greater than average risk due to the large number of health issues that are associated with having high blood pressure. Cases of heart failure, kidney failure, and stroke are on the rise and it is thought that such conditions are directly linked to high blood pressure and in turn an unhealthy diet. Medical professionals have therefore been working for years on dietary strategies for recovering normal blood pressure levels. The DASH diet is a result of this work with DASH standing for **D**ietary **A**pproaches to **S**topping **H**ypertension and focuses more on overall health than simply weight loss alone.

Hypertension (blood pressure) is calculated by measuring the pressure put on blood vessels and organs as blood is forced through the body. Blood pressure is measured by analysing both **Diastolic** pressure and **Systolic** pressure. **Diastolic** pressure is the measure of pressure within the veins between heartbeats, when the heart is at rest. **Systolic** pressure is the measure of pressure in the veins whilst the heart beats. By correlating these two numbers medical professional are able to provide accurate blood pressure readings. The DASH diet has been proven to lower blood pressure in both healthy individuals and those suffering from hypertension.

The DASH diet is a trusted, tested and tasty dieting strategy which is recommended by many medical professionals, nutritional experts and the health conscious worldwide. The fact is our health is massively affected by what we eat and the right change in diet can be nothing short of life changing. In my role as a nutritional coach, I regularly recommended the DASH diet and have witnessed the transformational effects that can happen when individuals eat plenty of the correct foods and throw in a bit of light exercise. Our blood pressure wants to behave; we just need to help it along a bit. We do this through the Dash diet by focussing on fruits, vegetables and lean proteins like chicken and fish whilst cutting down the red meats, processed sugars, salt, and unhelpful fats.

Not only does the DASH diet lower blood pressure, assist in weight loss and help to prevent illnesses like heart disease it also, due to the high amounts of fruits and vegetables lower the risk of developing diabetes and even cancers. Lowering blood pressure naturally without drugs is an attractive proposition to most of us and if we can do so whilst enjoying familiar whole foods it quickly becomes more so. This inexpensive combination of dietary techniques ultimately culminates in one of the most highly praised dieting strategies around and so if you'd like to lose weight whilst lowering high blood pressure and to do so without counting the calories, well then, The DASH diet is definitely for you!

DASH Diet: The Complete Beginners Guide to Dash Dieting, including Meal Plan and Recipes for Weight Loss and Clean Eating has written with the beginner in mind and was designed to be the ideal go-to guide for anyone aiming for a healthier future. First of all, we will cover the key steps and features of the DASH diet along with corresponding health benefits. Once we have a solid understanding of the DASH diet the two-week meal plan will ensure you get the best possible start on your journey to lowering blood pressure naturally (results can be seen in as little as 2-4 weeks). The book ends with a collection of delicious DASH-friendly recipes that have been chosen not only for their health benefits but also for flavour, simplicity to prepare, and prep time. I trust the information compiled within this book will prove useful to you years to come, I wish you long life and good health. It's now time DASH towards a healthier life.

Ensure that Meals are Fulfilling

The feeling of being full after a meal is defined as being satiated and satiety is known to suppress the feeling of hunger for longer. When we eat and drink our bodies produce a number of different chemicals and signal as the food/drink is digested, this is why we feel 'full' or satiated after a healthy meal. So, what do we need to do in order to enhance feelings of satiety and gain greater of control over feelings of hunger?

- Generally speaking, foods that are high in protein make us feel 'fuller for longer' so try to include some protein at least every other meal throughout the day.

- Alcohol stimulates and magnifies appetite especially in the short-term, let alone the effect it has on even the very best of intentions therefor alcoholic beverages for DASH dieters is a no-no.

- Limit 'liquid calories' by keeping sugary drinks to an absolute minimum. Cut them out altogether if you can and that most definitely includes coffee.

- Paying closer attention to your food while you eat and chewing each bite for longer are both known to increase feelings of satiety.

- Try to eat more meals that are high in water like soups. These allow us to keep our usual portion size while lowering the overall calorie content of the meal.

- Prepping meals from scratch allows for greater control over what we eat and when.

Reduce Your Sodium Intake

The human body requires **sodium** to stay alive. It's needed to maintain balanced levels of hydration, contact and relax muscles and even transmit nerve signals and impulses. However, it doesn't take much sodium to overdo it and the sodium levels contained within our daily salt intake are where a lot of high blood pressure issues start. Less sodium in your diet can help lower hypertension or even completely avoid blood pressure related conditions.

In the original DASH diet research, sodium intake was lowered to 1 teaspoon daily. Over time this can usually be lowered to around 2/3 of a teaspoon. Lowering your salt/sodium is really simple, below are some simple ideas to get you started:

- ALWAYS read the label.

- Create your own personalised meal plan.

- Prep your own meals.

- Try out different spices.

- Cut of junk food.

- Eat fresh foods.
- Cut out canned foods.

Increase Magnesium, Calcium and Potassium Intake

Magnesium, calcium, and potassium play extremely important roles in the proper functioning of our bodies. Minerals, nutrients and are known as electrolytes (along with other minerals) and together they help regulate many of the body's functions including bone and muscle development alongside maintaining nerve and heart signals. Throughout the day we lose electrolytes by sweating and going to the bathroom and so it is important to replenish them at regular intervals and drink plenty of water. Three of the most important electrolytes are:

- **Magnesium** aids nerve function, bone and strength development, and also helps to keep up a healthy and proper heart rhythm.
- **Calcium** helps with bone development, muscle contractions, blood clotting, and even cell division.
- **Potassium** helps to maintain stable blood pressure levels as well as heart contractions and muscles function.

When we are lacking in magnesium, calcium, and potassium we face electrolyte imbalances which could lead to the following symptoms:

- Muscle cramps.
- General feelings of weakness.
- Anxiety.
- Unstable blood pressure levels.
- Body fluid imbalance.
- Short term illnesses like cold/flu.
- Joint pain.
- Trouble concentrating.
- Heart palpitations.
- Insomnia.
- Higher than usual temperature/fever.
- Constant thirst.
- Headaches/Migraines.
- Dizziness.
- Tiredness.
- Twitches.

To increase your intake of magnesium, calcium, potassium and other minerals and electrolytes we must eat at least 4 portions of fruit and at least 5 portions of different vegetables each day. Eating citrus at least 3 times a week will provide a potassium boost and for extra magnesium, potassium, calcium, and fibre look no further than peas or nuts and seeds. When choosing dairy products (for calcium) ensure to choose products with the lowest fat content possible.

Increase Your Fibre Intake

Dietary fibre is well documented as being a crucial part of any diet, with the recommended daily allowance (RDA) being between 22g and 38g. However, when adding extra fibre to our diets it is important that it is done gradually because is we overdo it and increase our fibre intake too much too soon it can cause us a number of problems, such as:

- Bloating.
- Constipation.
- Diarrhea.
- Abdominal pain.
- Intestinal blockages.
- Low blood sugar levels.

Signs that you're increasing fibre too fast include:

- A change in bowel movements.
- Stomach ache/abdominal pain.
- A bloated or gassy feeling.
- Mineral deficiencies.

A final word to remember is that when we eat fibre it is important to drink plenty of water to aid the digestion process.

Find replacements for those sweet tooth cravings

It's extremely common to have 'sweet tooth' cravings after a meal (don't I know it!) but thanks to these healthy treats these cravings can be satiated without reaching for the chocolate:

- Any piece of fresh fruit contains enough natural sugars to satisfy sugary cravings.
- A spoonful of natural honey should curb those sugar cravings.
- Frozen grapes or cherries are great sweet treats full of antioxidants.
- Trail mix.
- Smoothies (homemade).
- Chewing gum.
- Wholegrain cinnamon raisin toast.
- Jam/jelly or fruit spread on crackers.

Reduce caffeine intake and drink lots of fluids

Caffeinated drinks are often packed with sugar and so it really is best to avoid them altogether when DASH dieting, however, if we must get our caffeine fix set a limit of 2 drinks per day at most. When possible choose decaffeinated low-sugar versions of your usual beverage.

The general advice is that we should drink 8 cups (or 3-1/2 pints) per day. Unfortunately, many of us find it difficult to keep up with our recommended water intake. Part of the reason for this is that our taste buds have gotten so used to sugary drinks that 'plain' water just doesn't appeal. I strongly suggest giving fresh water a chance as after only a day or two it is clear that water satiates thirst to a much greater extent than its highly caffeinated and sugar-packed counterparts.

- Keeping a water jug on your desk is a great way to remind yourself to stay hydrated.

- When carrying a bag, always pack a bottle of water.

- Keep a fresh bottle of water in your car at all times.

- Start each morning with a large cup of water.

- Drink at least 1 cup of water with every meal.

Nuts are a perfect snack

Nuts are extremely healthy, filling, and 100% natural which makes them an ideal snack for DASH dieters. Nuts are a great source of healthy fats, protein and are rich in anti-oxidants as well as being packed with other nutrients. Just a small handful of nuts can boost energy levels for hours and work perfectly for pre/post workout or even midnight snack. Nuts may not be the most appetising of foods and we must avoid the flavoured varieties that carry large amounts of salts and other additives but nuts cannot be overlooked, the healthy oils, fats and vitamins like E and B6 which are common in nuts are often rarely found in other foods and are important for everything from bone development and proper brain function. For vegetarians nuts are a welcome source of protein, however, all nuts are different, some are packed full of calcium whilst others are rich in anti-oxidants, so here's a brief rundown of some of the more 'everyday' varieties:

- Walnuts in particular are known for having the highest levels of anti-oxidants and omega-3 which means they are ideal for sufferers of inflammatory conditions and they even help prevent cellular damage which could result in cancer and even heart failure.

- Cashews contain plenty of iron which helps prevent anaemic conditions whilst the high zinc content boosts the immune system and works towards maintaining healthy vision. Cashews also boast bumper levels magnesium which is great for cognitive functions like memory.

- Pecans are perfect for lowering cholesterol and have been proven to contain almost as many anti-oxidants as walnuts.

- Pistachios carry around 2 calories per nut, so this makes them a Dash dieter's dream, full of potassium and vitamin B6 which are proven to elevate moods and even ward of lung cancer.

- Eating just 1 brazil nut provides you with your entire daily requirement of selenium, be to limit yourself to one or two portions daily as too much selenium can be hazardous to health. Brazil nuts can even help prevent conditions like breast and bone cancer.

- Almonds contain high levels of calcium which makes them an ideal snack for non-dairy eaters

- Hazelnuts are a great source of folate which helps to regulate the homocysteine within the body which is an amino acid known to be linked to numerous heart conditions as well as Parkinson's disease.

14 Day Meal Plan and Recipe Guide

The typical DASH diet menu should average at around 1600 calories daily and include at least four portions of vegetables and two portions of fruit as well as the following:

- 5-6 oz. (141g-170g) whole grains
- 1 oz. (28g) nuts and seeds
- 1 tablespoon of healthy oils such as safflower, canola or olive
- 2 servings of low-fat dairy products
- 5 oz. (141g-170g)

Primarily the DASH consists of fruits, vegetables, whole grains, and some low-fat dairy, fish, lean meats, poultry, and plenty of nuts/seeds and beans for all of which contain healthy fats and nutrients. The following meal plans will get your DASH off to the best possible start and were designed to keep you feeling satiated for longer, cutting out the need for mid-morning and afternoon snacks (if you feel hungry grab a handful of nuts or a piece of fruit).

Day 1
Breakfast
Cinnamon and Oatmeal Gingerbreads, half an Apple and a glass of Water

Ingredients (4 servings)
1 ½ cup of coarse or steel cut oatmeal
1 teaspoon of cinnamon
¼ teaspoon of cloves
¼ teaspoon of ginger
¼ teaspoon of cardamom
¼ teaspoon of allspice
1 tablespoon of honey
Water as specified by coarse oatmeal packet cooking instructions
Method
1. Cook the coarse oatmeal as specified on its packaging and mix in all of the spices whilst cooking.
2. Once the coarse oatmeal is cooked, mix in the honey and leave to cool.

Serving your Cinnamon and Oatmeal Gingerbreads
Just snap off a piece of this breakfast treat and be on your way. Ideal for travel and lasts at least 3 days if properly stored.

Sesame Prawn Stir Fry and a glass of Water

Ingredients (2 servings)
350g fresh prawns
2 cloves of garlic, grated
1 large white onion, chopped
1 squash, chopped
2 cups shitake mushrooms
1 red bell pepper, chopped
4 tablespoons liquid aminos
2 teaspoons sesame oil
2 tablespoon hemp seeds
1 tablespoon honey
Olive oil

Method

1. Heat 1 tablespoon of olive oil in a frying pan or skillet over a medium-high heat.
2. Add the prawns to the frying pan and cook for 3 minutes turning midway. Remove the frying pan from the heat and put the prawns to one side.
3. Whilst the prawns cook whisk together the sesame oil, Aminos liquid, honey and hemp seeds.
4. Heat 1 tablespoon of olive oil in a wok or large frying pan over a medium heat.
5. Add the garlic and onions to the frying pan and cook for 2 minutes before throwing in the rest of the vegetables and stir-frying for 5 minutes.

6. Pour the sauce into the pan and cook for a
    further 2-3 minutes.

Serving your Sesame Prawn Stir Fry
Serve with quinoa or brown rice.

Zahtar Salmon with Citrus, Green leaf Salad and Sparkling Mineral Water

Ingredients (2 servings)
2 salmon fillets
1 ½ teaspoons of Zahtar spice
1 clove of garlic finely chopped
1 teaspoon of dried coriander
1 tablespoon of lemon juice
Salt and ground black pepper to taste
Olive oil
Mixed green leaves
1 tomato, sliced
1 carrot, peeled and cut julienne
Vinaigrette of choice

Method

1. Mix the zahtar, coriander, lemon juice, garlic, 1 tablespoon of olive oil and a little salt and ground black pepper to taste in a bowl.
2. Place the salmon fillets in the mix, coat thoroughly, cover and place in the fridge for at least 30 minutes.
3. Warm a little oil in a pan over a medium heat.
4. Gently place the salmon fillets in the pan skin side down, pour any remaining marinade mix over the salmon and cook for 4-6minutes, carefully turning midway.
5. Toss together the mixed green leaves, sliced tomato, carrot slices and some salt and pepper to taste and a little of your chosen vinaigrette.

Serving your Zahtar Salmon with Citrus and Green Leaf Salad
Serve hot atop a bed of salad.

Day 2
Breakfast
Salmon and Avocado on Toast with a glass of Water

Ingredients
Bread (gluten-free), toasted
1 avocado, sliced
1 packet of smoked salmon
¼ cup finely chopped radish sprouts
Salt and ground black pepper
Lemon juice
Method
1. Top the toast with salmon and radish sprouts.

Serving your Salmon and Avocado on Toast
Serve with a little salt and ground black pepper along with a dash of lemon juice.

Lunch
Quinoa Salad and a glass of Water

Ingredients (2 servings)
1 cup of quinoa
1 white onion, finely chopped
2 carrots, roughly chopped
2 parsnips, roughly chopped
1 teaspoon thyme
Tahini dressing
Salt and ground black pepper
Olive oil
Method
1. Coat the carrots, parsnips, and onion with a little olive oil and sprinkle over the thyme.
2. Place the carrots, parsnips, and onion on a parchment lined baking tray and into a pre-heated oven at 425°F/200°C (gas mark 7), cook for 25-30 minutes turning midway.
3. Whilst the vegetables roast, cook the quinoa as per the instructions on the pack.
4. Once cooked add the roasted vegetables to the quinoa and mix well.

Serving your Quinoa Salad
Serve hot with a dollop of tahini dressing.

Bulgur Stuffed Mushrooms with sparkling mineral water

Ingredients

4-6 portabella mushrooms washed with stalks removed and hollowed out
1 cup bulgur wheat
800ml chicken stock
200ml chicken stock
1 red bell pepper, diced
1 red onion finely chopped
4 cloves of garlic finely chopped
1 ½ inch piece of ginger, grated
½ teaspoon cayenne pepper
½ teaspoon cumin
½ teaspoon turmeric
½ teaspoon paprika
1 teaspoon dried basil
Salt and ground black pepper
1 teaspoon of sugar
1 packet of dried apricots, finely chopped
Olive oil

Method

1. Cook the bulgur wheat as instructed by the packet.
2. Heat some olive oil in a large pan over a medium heat.
3. Throw the onions into the pan, lower to a medium heat and cook for 2 minutes.
4. Dice the mushroom stalks and add them to the pan along with the rest of the peppers and all of

the herbs and spices. Stir well and cook for 3
minutes.

5. When the bulgur wheat is cooked mix it with
    the vegetable mix and gently stuff the
    mushroom caps with the mix.
6. Cook in the oven on a medium heat for 15-
    18minutes.
7. In a small saucepan pour the 200ml chicken
    stock along with the dried apricots and sugar
    and place on a medium-low heat.
8. Gently crush the apricots with the back of a
    spoon whilst cooking, stir throughout, until the
    liquids have reduced by half.

Serving your Bulgur stuffed Mushrooms
Serve hot with steamed kale or fresh green leaf salad.

Day 3
Breakfast
Hard Boiled Egg and Tomato Juice

Ingredients
Eggs (cook more than one and keep them for another day)
Water
Method
1. Heat a pan of water over a medium heat, bring to the boil and simmer.
2. Gently place the eggs into the water and cook for 6 minutes for runny centres and 7 for cooked through.
3. Remove the eggs from the water and immediately place them in cold water to cool.

Serving your Hard Boiled Eggs
Peel and serve with a glass of fresh tomato juice.

Mixed Peppers and Spinach Frittatas

Ingredients
100g spinach leaves
1 red bell pepper, diced
1 yellow bell pepper, diced
1 onion, chopped
6 large eggs
1 ½ teaspoons garam masala
Salt and ground black pepper to taste
½ cup of cheddar cheese
Method
1. Heat some oil in a large frying pan over a medium heat.
2. Throw the onions into the frying pan and sweat for 3 minutes or until soft.
3. Add the chopped peppers to the frying pan and cook for a further 3-5 minutes.
4. Mix the eggs and cheese and a little salt and ground black pepper to taste in a large mixing bowl or jug. When thoroughly mixed pour the mix onto the eggs and cook for 3 minutes
5. Top with an extra sprinkling of cheese and place the frying pan under the grill and cook for a further 5 minutes or until the frittata begins to brown.

Serving your Mixed Peppers and Spinach Frittatas
Cut into quarters and serve with a mixed green leaf salad.

Pan Seared Wild Salmon with Broccoli and Asparagus, Brown Rice and a large glass of Water

Ingredients
2-4 skinless/deboned wild salmon fillets
1 cup sliced shitake mushrooms
½ tablespoon lemon juice
½ tablespoon lime juice
½ teaspoon medium-heat chili flakes
1 tablespoon black pepper
Salt to taste
½ tablespoon chopped chives
½ tablespoon parsley
125g asparagus tips
1 large cup of broccoli florets
Olive oil

Method
1. Heat 1 tablespoon of olive oil in a large frying pan or skillet over a medium heat.
2. Add the chili flakes and cook for 30 seconds.
3. Coat the top side of the salmon with black pepper, place into the frying pan and cook for 3-4 minutes before carefully turning and cooking for a further 2-3 minutes.
4. Whilst the salmon cooks steam the broccoli and asparagus tips for 6-8 minutes.
5. Remove the salmon from the frying pan and pour over the lemon and lime juices.

Serving your Pan Seared Salmon with Broccoli and Asparagus
Garnish with chives and parsley, serve hot with brown rice or quinoa.

Day 4
Breakfast
Mango, Ginger and Pineapple Smoothie

Ingredients
1 cup of pineapple chunks
1 cup of mango chunks
½ cucumber, peeled and roughly chopped
1 banana, peeled and chopped into chunks
½ cup of ice cubes
½ teaspoon of freshly grated ginger
¼ teaspoon of cinnamon
¼ teaspoon of turmeric
5-8 mint leaves
½ cup of green tea cooled
½ cup of water
Method
1. Place all of the ingredients into a food processor or blender and blend until smooth.

Serving your Mango, Ginger and Pineapple Smoothie
Serve immediately in a tall glass with a sprinkling of chia seeds.

Beetroot Salad with Sparkling Mineral Water

Ingredients
1 ½ beetroot, grated or chopped julienne
1 carrot, grated or chopped julienne
1 pear, diced
1 apple, diced
1 clove garlic, grated or minced
1 cup mixed green leaves
1 tablespoon almonds
1 tablespoon hemp oil
Method
1. In a large mixing bowl mix together the beetroot, carrot, pear, apple, garlic, almonds and hemp oil.

Serving your Beetroot Salad
Serve immediately atop a bed of mixed green leaves.

Garlic, Chili and Ginger Cod Loin with Green Leaves and a glass of Water

Ingredients (2-4 servings)
2-4 cod loin fillets
3 cloves of garlic finely chopped
1-inch piece of ginger, grated
½ teaspoon of dried chili flakes
1 tablespoon of lemon juice
2 tablespoons of olive oil
Salt and ground black pepper to taste
Mixed green leaves
1 tomato, sliced
1 carrot, peeled and cut julienne

Method
1. Mix all of the ingredients and fully coat the cod loins ensuring they are evenly covered.
2. Heat some oil in a pan.
3. In a bowl toss the mixed green leaves, sliced tomato and carrot into a bowl.
4. Place the cod loins skin down in the pan, along with any remaining marinade and cook for 2-3 minutes or until the skin is crisp.
5. Gently turn the cod loins and cook for a further 2-3 minutes.

Serving your Garlic, Chili and Ginger Cod Loin with Green Leaves
Serve your cod loins hot atop a bed of salad.

Day 5
Breakfast
Eat your Greens Detox Smoothie

Ingredients (4 servings)
4 golden delicious apples, cored
2 pears, cored
2 cucumbers
1 cup of spinach
1 cup kale
½ a lemon
½ a lime
4 sticks of celery
1 teaspoon grated ginger root
Ground black pepper to taste (optional)
1 cup ice
Method
1.   Blend or juice all of the ingredients.

Serving your Eat your Greens Detox Smoothie
Serve immediately.

Smoked Salmon and Potato Rosti an apple and a glass of water

Ingredients

I large russet or Maris Piper potato
1 tablespoon of butter
110g soft goat cheese chopped into small cubes
Thinly sliced smoked salmon
1 clove of garlic, grated
2 teaspoons of freshly grated ginger
Zest of ½ a lemon
¼ red onion, finely chopped
½ a tomato, chopped
1 large handful of chopped spinach leaves

Method- Rosti

1. Peel the potato and grate into a bowl.
2. Rinse the grated potato with water to remove any excess starch and then squeeze the potato hard in your hands to remove any liquids.
3. Season the potato with salt and ground black pepper.
4. Place the butter in a frying pan or skillet and melt over a medium heat.
5. Whilst the butter melts, using your hands shape the potato into a round 'burger' shape.
6. Place the potato in the frying pan or skillet and cook for 16-18 minutes turning midway.
7. Once cooked place your potato rosti to one side.

Method- Topping

1. In a bowl, mix the goat cheese, spinach leaves, onion, tomato, garlic, lemon zest, ginger and a little salt and ground black pepper to taste.

Serving your Smoked Salmon and Potato Rosti

Spoon some of the topping mix on to the rostie and place a couple of layers of smoked salmon on top, serve warm.

Dinner
Tomato and Herb Seabass

Ingredients (2-4 servings)
2-4 sea bass fillets
1 packet of sun-dried tomatoes, chopped
1 handful of cherry tomatoes, chopped
½ teaspoon of dried basil
1 teaspoon of mixed herbs
2 tablespoon tomato puree
2 cloves of garlic finely chopped
½ white onion, finely chopped
Salt and ground black pepper to taste
150g spinach leaves
Method
1. Mix the sun-dried tomatoes, cherry tomatoes and crush them with the back of a spoon.
2. Add the mixed herbs, basil, tomato puree, garlic, onions, salt and ground black pepper.
3. Coat the seabass in the tomato and herb marinade, cover and refrigerate for at least 2 hours.
4. Preheat the oven to 400°F/200°C (gas mark 6).
5. Place the sea bass in a ceramic dish along with the marinade sauce and cook for 15 minutes.

Serving your Tomato and Herb Seabass
Serve hot atop a bed of fresh spinach leaves.

Day 6
Breakfast
Gluten Free Breakfast Crepes with a glass of Water

Ingredients
1 cup multi-purpose gluten-free flour
2 eggs
1 teaspoon vanilla essence
1 cup semi-skimmed milk
Coconut oil
¼ raspberries
¼ cup blueberries
Method
1. Whisk together the eggs, vanilla essence, almond milk and water until combined.
2. Gradually add the flour to the mix, whisking throughout.
3. Heat 2 tablespoons of coconut oil in a frying pan over a medium heat, once melted add to the batter mix.
4. Heat 1 tablespoon of coconut oil in the frying pan over a medium heat and pour in between ¼ and ½ cup of the pancake batter into the frying pan.
5. Cook the pancake for 2-3 minutes turning midway.
6. Repeat for the rest of the pancake batter mix.

Serving your Gluten Free Pancakes
Serve immediately with mixed berries.

Lunch
Ham Salad

Ingredients
1 slice of thick cut ham
4 cups lettuce
½ a cucumber
2 cups spinach
2 tomatoes, chopped
¼ cup sliced radish
½ cup grated carrot
½ cup chopped red onion
Method
1. Toss all of the vegetables in a bowl, drizzle over a little olive oil and a little salt and pepper.

Serving your Ham Salad
Serve immediately alongside the ham.

Light Spice Butternut Squash and Lentil Stew

Ingredients
3 cups of butternut squash chopped and cooked
½ cup lentils
½ cup red lentils
1 cup of carrots, chopped
1 red onion, chopped
½ cup of broccoli, chopped
2 cloves of garlic, finely chopped
½ inch piece of fresh ginger, grated
800ml vegetable stock
½ teaspoon of turmeric
½ teaspoon of medium curry powder
1 tablespoon of olive oil
Ground black pepper to taste

Method- Butternut squash

1. Chop the butternut squash and mix it in a bowl with a little olive oil, and pepper.

2. Place the butternut squash on a baking and into the oven at 190°F, cook for 20 minutes.

Method- Light Spice Butternut Squash and Lentil Stew

1. Heat the olive oil in a large cooking pot over a medium-high heat.

2. Add the onions to the pot and cook for 3 minutes.

3. Add the garlic and ginger to the pot and cook for a further 2 minutes.

4. Stir in the carrots, lentils, curry powder, turmeric, vegetable stock and bring to the boil, then reduce the heat and cook for 10-12 minutes.
5. Add the broccoli, butternut squash and a little salt and pepper to taste to the stew and cook for a further 10 minutes.

Serving your Light Spice Butternut Squash and Lentil Stew
Serve in serving bowls (4 servings) with a sprinkling of grated cheese.

Day 7
Breakfast
Spinach Bruschetta

Ingredients
Bruschetta
1 cup of spinach
½ red onion, minced
1 clove of garlic
Olive oil
½ cup Greek yogurt
1 tablespoon fresh mint
Salt and ground black pepper to taste
¼ cup chopped walnuts
Method
1. Drizzle some olive oil over the bruschetta and place it in the oven for 5 minutes.
2. Whilst the bruschetta is toasting, boil the spinach for 3-5 minutes before draining off.
3. Heat some olive oil in a pan and sauté the onions and garlic for 3 minutes.
4. Mix the spinach, onions, garlic, yoghurt, walnuts, and mint in a bowl.

Serving your Spinach Bruschetta
Serve the toasted bruschetta topped with the spinach mix.

Lunch
Roasted Curry Cauliflower and Flax Seeds

Ingredients
3 cups broccoli florets
2 tablespoons flax seeds
2 cloves of garlic, grated
2 tablespoon lime juice
1 tablespoon lemon juice
2 tablespoons curry powder
1 tablespoon olive oil
Salt and ground black pepper to taste

Method
1. In a bowl whisk together the olive oil, garlic and curry powder before coating the cauliflower with the mix.
2. Place the cauliflower on a parchment lined baking tray, into a pre-heated oven at 400°F/200°C (gas mark 6) and cook for 14-16 minutes.
3. Add the flax seeds and a little salt and pepper to taste and cook for a further 10 minutes.
4. Remove the cauliflower from the oven and drizzle with the lemon and limes juices.

Serving your Roasted Curry Cauliflower and Flax Seeds
Serve hot with brown rice.

Dinner
Garlic, Chili and Ginger Cod Loin with Green Leaves

Ingredients
2-4 cod loin fillets
3 cloves of garlic finely chopped
1-inch piece of ginger, grated
½ teaspoon of dried chili flakes
1 tablespoon of lemon juice
2 tablespoons of olive oil
Salt and ground black pepper to taste
Mixed green leaves
1 tomato, sliced
1 carrot, peeled and cut julienne
Method
1. Mix all of the ingredients and fully coat the cod loins ensuring they are evenly covered.
2. Heat some oil in a pan.
3. In a bowl toss the mixed green leaves, sliced tomato and carrot into a bowl.
4. Place the cod loins skin down in the pan, along with any remaining marinade and cook for 2-3 minutes or until the skin is crisp.
5. Gently turn the cod loins and cook for a further 2-3 minutes.

Serving your Garlic, Chili and Ginger Cod Loin with Green Leaves
Serve your cod loins hot atop a bed of salad.

Day 8
Breakfast
Hard Boiled Egg and Tomato Juice

Ingredients
Eggs (cook more than one and keep them for another day)
Water
Method
1. Heat a pan of water over a medium heat, bring to the boil and simmer.
2. Gently place the eggs into the water and cook for 6 minutes for runny centres and 7 for cooked through.
3. Remove the eggs from the water and immediately place them in cold water to cool.

Serving your Hard Boiled Eggs
Peel and serve with a glass of fresh tomato juice.

Lunch
Bacon and Cheese Frittatas

Ingredients
1 pack of smoked bacon, roughly chopped
1 cup of grated cheddar cheese
½ cup chopped spinach leaves
6 large eggs
Salt and black pepper to taste
Olive oil
Method
1. Heat some olive oil in a large frying pan and fry the bacon over a medium-high heat for 3-4 minutes turning midway pour away and excess fats.
2. Whilst the bacon is cooking mix the eggs, cheese, spinach and a little salt and pepper to taste in a large mixing bowl.
3. Pour the eggs and cheese mixture over the bacon and cook for 3 minutes.
4. Top with an extra sprinkling of cheese and place the frying pan under the grill and cook for a further 5 minutes or until the frittata begins to brown.

Serving your Bacon and Cheese Frittatas
Serve hot with a green leaf salad.

Dinner
Sesame Prawn Stir Fry

Ingredients
450g fresh prawns
2 cloves of garlic, grated
1 large white onion, chopped
1 squash, chopped
2 cups shitake mushrooms
1 red bell pepper, chopped
4 tablespoons liquid aminos
2 teaspoons sesame oil
2 tablespoon hemp seeds
2 tablespoon honey
Olive oil

Method

1. Heat 1 tablespoon of olive oil in a frying pan or skillet over a medium-high heat.

2. Add the prawns to the frying pan and cook for 3 minutes turning midway. Remove the frying pan from the heat and put the prawns to one side.

3. Whilst the prawns cook whisk together the sesame oil, Aminos liquid, honey and hemp seeds.

4. Heat 1 tablespoon of olive oil in a wok or large frying pan over a medium heat.

5. Add the garlic and onions to the frying pan and cook for 2 minutes before throwing in the rest of the vegetables and stir-frying for 5 minutes.

6. Pour the sauce into the pan and cook for a further 2-3 minutes.

Serving your Sesame Prawn Stir Fry
Serve with quinoa or brown rice.

Day 9
Breakfast
Salmon and Avocado on Toast with a glass of Water

Ingredients
Bread (gluten-free), toasted
1 avocado, sliced
1 packet of smoked salmon
¼ cup finely chopped radish sprouts
Salt and ground black pepper
Lemon juice
Method
1. Top the toast with salmon and radish sprouts.

Serving your Salmon and Avocado on Toast
Serve with a little salt and ground black pepper along with a dash of lemon juice.

Lunch
Ham Salad

Ingredients
1 slice of thick cut ham
4 cups lettuce
½ a cucumber
2 cups spinach
2 tomatoes, chopped
¼ cup sliced radish
½ cup grated carrot
½ cup chopped red onion
Method
1. Toss all of the vegetables in a bowl, drizzle over a little olive oil and a little salt and pepper.

Serving your Ham Salad
Serve immediately alongside the ham.

Dinner
Salmon Chowder

Ingredients
1 large salmon fillet
¼ cup chopped carrot
¼ cup chopped celery
1 cup instant mash potato flakes
2 tablespoons chives, finely chopped
800ml chicken broth
2 cup cauliflower
¼ cup chopped dill
1 teaspoon dried tarragon
1 teaspoon mustard
Salt and ground black pepper to taste
Olive oil
Method
1. Heat some olive oil in a large saucepan over a medium heat.
2. Throw the carrot and the celery into the pan and cook for 3 minutes before adding the chicken stock and bringing to the boil.
3. Add the cauliflower, water, chives, and salmon and bring to the simmer for 8 minutes.
4. Remove the salmon fillet and break it apart using a fork before returning it to the mix along with the instant potato flakes, dill, tarragon, mustard and a little salt and pepper.
5. Cook on a low heat for 3-5 minutes, storing throughout.

Serving your Salmon Chowder

Serve hot with a side salad.

Day 10
Breakfast
Eat your Greens Detox Smoothie

Ingredients (4 servings)
4 golden delicious apples, cored
2 pears, cored
2 cucumbers
1 cup of spinach
1 cup kale
½ a lemon
½ a lime
4 sticks of celery
1 teaspoon grated ginger root
Ground black pepper to taste (optional)
1 cup ice
Method
1.   Blend or juice all of the ingredients.

Serving your Eat your Greens Detox Smoothie
Serve immediately.

Bulgur Stuffed Mushrooms

Ingredients
4-6 portabella mushrooms, washed with stalks removed and hollowed out (serves 4)
1 cup bulgur wheat
800ml chicken stock
200ml chicken stock
1 red bell pepper, diced
1 red onion finely chopped
4 cloves of garlic finely chopped
1 ½ inch piece of ginger, grated
½ teaspoon cayenne pepper
½ teaspoon cumin
½ teaspoon turmeric
½ teaspoon paprika
1 teaspoon dried basil
Salt and ground black pepper
1 teaspoon of sugar
1 packet of dried apricots, finely chopped
Olive oil

Method
1. Cook the bulgur wheat as instructed by the packet.
2. Heat some olive oil in a large pan over a medium heat.
3. Throw the onions into the pan, lower to a medium heat and cook for 2 minutes.
4. Dice the mushroom stalks and add them to the pan along with the rest of the peppers and all of

the herbs and spices. Stir well and cook for 3
minutes.

5.   When the bulgur wheat is cooked mix it with
     the vegetable mix and gently stuff the
     mushroom caps with the mix.
6.   Cook in the oven on a medium heat for 15-
     18minutes.
7.   In a small saucepan pour the200ml chicken
     stock along with the dried apricots and sugar
     and place on a medium-low heat.
8.   Gently crush the apricots with the back of a
     spoon whilst cooking, stir throughout, until the
     liquids have reduced by half.

Serving your Bulgur stuffed Mushrooms
Serve hot with steamed kale or fresh green leaf salad.

Dinner
**Herb Crusted Cod with Steamed Vegetables and a
Large Glass of Water**

Ingredients
Cod loins (approx. 3oz per portion)
Mixed herbs
Chilli flakes
1 tbl spoon lime juice
½ cup brown rice
½ cup fine green beans
½ cup broccoli
½ cup of carrots
Method
1. Mix the herbs, chilli flakes, and lime juice. Fully coat the cod loins ensuring they are evenly covered.
2. Heat some oil in a pan.
3. Place the broccoli, carrots and green beans into the steamer and cook for 8 minutes.
4. Place the cod loins skin down in the pan, along with any remaining marinade and cook for 2-3 minutes or until the skin is crisp.
5. Gently turn the cod loins and cook for a further 2-3 minutes.

Serving your Herb Crusted Cod with Steamed Vegetables and a Large Glass of Water
Serve immediately.

Day 11
Breakfast
Salmon and Avocado on Toast with a glass of Water

Ingredients

Bread (gluten-free), toasted
1 avocado, sliced
1 packet of smoked salmon
¼ cup finely chopped radish sprouts
Salt and ground black pepper
Lemon juice
Method
1. Top the toast with salmon and radish sprouts.

Serving your Salmon and Avocado on Toast
Serve with a little salt and ground black pepper along with a dash of lemon juice.

Single Pot Quinoa Broccoli

Ingredients
3 cups broccoli florets
1 cup quinoa
1 onion, finely chopped
3 cloves of garlic, grated
1 shallot, finely chopped
800ml vegetable stock
1 tablespoon balsamic vinegar
2 teaspoons Italian mixed herbs
Salt and ground black pepper to taste
1 tablespoon olive oil
1 cup grated cheese of choice (optional)
Method
1. Heat some olive oil in a saucepan over a medium heat. Throw the onions, garlic, shallot, balsamic vinegar and Italian mixed herbs into the saucepan and cook for 3 minutes.
2. Add the quinoa to the saucepan along with a little salt and ground black pepper to taste, cook for 1-2 minutes before pouring the vegetable stock into the saucepan, cover and cook for 10 minutes.
3. Add the broccoli to the pan, replace the cover and cook over a low heat for a further 8-10 minutes.

Serving your Single Pot Quinoa Broccoli
Stir in the grated cheese and serve immediately.

Dinner
Ginger Beef and Broccoli Stir-Fry

Ingredients

500g sirloin beef steak cut into thin slices
2 cups of broccoli florets
1 cup of green beans, chopped
1 onion, chopped
1 medium-sized carrot, peeled and sliced julienne
1 cup of kale leaves, washed and chopped
2 garlic cloves, finely chopped
1 red pepper, sliced
1 teaspoon of turmeric
½ inch piece of fresh ginger, grated
2 tablespoons of wheat free tamari
1 tablespoon of fresh lemon juice
½ teaspoon of salt
½ teaspoon of ground black pepper
1 tablespoon of apple cider vinegar
1 ½ tablespoons of coconut oil

Method

1. Warm a frying pan over a medium-high heat, toss in and melt the coconut oil.

2. Add the garlic, red pepper, ginger and onion to the pan. Cook for 5-6 minutes.

3. Stir the beef slices into the pan and cook for a further 5-6 minutes.

4. Add the Turmeric, lemon juice, salt, pepper, carrot, kale leaves, broccoli, green beans and apple cider vinegar to the pan.

5. Stir well and cook over a medium heat for 13-15 minutes.

Serving your Ginger Beef and Broccoli Stir-Fry
Serve with brown rice and green leaf salad.
Day 12
Breakfast
Bagel with Peanut Butter and an Orange

Ingredients
Whole Wheat Bagels (1 per serving)
Low salt peanut butter
1 fresh orange
Serving your Bagel with Peanut Butter and an Orange
Simply spread 1 generous tablespoon of peanut butter on each half of the sliced bagel.

Lunch
5 Minute Salad

Ingredients

4 cups lettuce

½ a cucumber

2 cups spinach

2 tomatoes, chopped

¼ cup black olives

1 cup grated carrot

½ cup chopped red onion

Method

1. Toss all of the vegetables in a bowl, drizzle over a little olive oil and a little salt and pepper.

Serving your 5 Minute Salad

Serve immediately, alone or with a gluten-free bread roll.

Dinner
Ginger Beef and Broccoli Stir-Fry

Ingredients
500g sirloin beef steak cut into thin slices (4 servings)
2 cups of broccoli florets
1 cup of green beans, chopped
1 red onion, chopped
1 medium-sized carrot, peeled and sliced julienne
1 cup of kale leaves, washed and chopped
2 garlic cloves, finely chopped
1 red pepper, sliced
½ teaspoon of turmeric
½ inch piece of fresh ginger, grated
2 tablespoons of wheat free tamari
1 tablespoon of fresh lime juice
½ teaspoon of ground black pepper
1 ½ tablespoons of olive oil

Method

1. Warm a frying pan over a medium-high heat, pour in the olive oil.
2. Add the garlic, red pepper, ginger and onion to the pan. Cook for 5-6 minutes.
3. Stir the beef slices into the pan and cook for a further 5-6 minutes.
4. Add the Turmeric, lime juice, pepper, carrot, kale leaves, broccoli, green beans.
5. Stir well and cook over a medium heat for 13-15 minutes.

Serving your Ginger Beef and Broccoli Stir-Fry
Serve with brown rice.

Day 13
Breakfast
Eat your Greens Detox Smoothie

Ingredients (4 servings)
4 golden delicious apples, cored
2 pears, cored
2 cucumbers
1 cup of spinach
1 cup kale
½ a lemon
½ a lime
4 sticks of celery
1 teaspoon grated ginger root
Ground black pepper to taste (optional)
1 cup ice
Method
1. Blend or juice all of the ingredients.

Serving your Eat your Greens Detox Smoothie
Serve immediately.

Lunch
Ham and Swiss Cheese Whole Wheat Roll/Sandwich

Ingredients
Sliced ham
Swiss cheese
Whole wheat bread/roll
1 handful of lettuce leaves

Serving your Ham and Swiss Cheese Whole Wheat Roll/Sandwich

Another simple one! Layer bread, ham, cheese topped with plenty of lettuce and serve with a large glass of water.

Dinner
Dry Rub Chicken, Baked Potato and Salad

Ingredients
Baked potato (1 per portion)
2 chicken breast (1 per portion)
1 teaspoon of garlic powder
1 teaspoon of ginger powder
1 teaspoon mustard powder
½ Teaspoon cumin
½ teaspoon turmeric
½ teaspoon fresh ground pepper
Mixed green leaves

Method
Dry Rub Chicken
1. Mix the spices together in a bowl.
2. Generously apply an even coating of the dry rub mix to the chicken and refrigerate for at least 2 hours.
3. Place the chicken under the grill and cook for 18-20 minutes or until charred, turning midway.

-Baked Potato
1. Wash potatoes, prick a few times with a fork and lightly coat with olive oil.
2. Pre-heat the oven to 210 C/420 F and place the potato on the middle shelf and cook for 50-60 minutes.

Serving your Dry Rub Chicken, Baked Potato and Salad
Serve hot with mixed green leaves and a knob of butter for the baked potato.

Day 14
Breakfast
Whole Wheat English Breakfast Muffin with Orange or Pineapple Juice

Ingredients
1 whole wheat muffin
Fresh juice of choice
Strawberry/raspberry jam
Serving your Whole Wheat English Breakfast Muffin with Orange or Pineapple Juice
Top the muffin with a spoonful of strawberry or raspberry jam and enjoy with a glass of juice.

Lunch
Asparagus and Potato Frittata

Ingredients
125g asparagus tips
200g Maris Piper or King Edward potatoes peeled and
roughly chopped (2 servings)
4 large eggs, beaten
1 red onion, chopped
¼ cup of grated cheddar cheese
¼ teaspoon dried rosemary
¼ Italian mixed herbs
Black pepper to taste
Method
1. Boil some water to the boil in a saucepan, add
   the potatoes, bring to the simmer and cook for
   10 minutes.
2. Add the asparagus tips to the saucepan and
   cook for a further 2-3 minutes.
3. Whilst the potatoes and asparagus cook, heat
   some oil in a large frying pan over a medium
   heat.
4. Throw the onions into the frying pan and sweat
   for 4-6 minutes or until soft.
5. Drain the asparagus and potatoes and put them
   to one side.
6. Mix the eggs, Italian mixed herbs, rosemary, a
   little black pepper to taste, and cheese in a large
   mixing bowl or jug, when thoroughly mixed
   pour the mix onto the onions.

7. Haphazardly add the asparagus and potatoes to the frying pan with the eggs, cheese, and onions, cook for 5-8 minutes.

8. Top with an extra sprinkling of cheese and place the frying pan under the grill and cook for a further 5-7 minutes or until the frittata begins to brown.

Serving your Asparagus and Potato Frittata
Cut into quarters and serve.

Dinner
Tomato and Herb Seabass

Ingredients (2-4 servings)
2-4 sea bass fillets
1 packet of sun-dried tomatoes, chopped
1 handful of cherry tomatoes, chopped
½ teaspoon of dried basil
1 teaspoon of mixed herbs
2 tablespoon tomato puree
2 cloves of garlic finely chopped
½ white onion, finely chopped
Salt and ground black pepper to taste
150g spinach leaves
Method
1. Mix the sun-dried tomatoes, cherry tomatoes and crush them with the back of a spoon.
2. Add the mixed herbs, basil, tomato puree, garlic, onions, salt and ground black pepper.
3. Coat the sea bass in the tomato and herb marinade, cover and refrigerate for at least 2 hours.
4. Preheat the oven to 400°F/200°C (gas mark 6).
5. Place the sea bass in a ceramic dish along with the marinade sauce and cook for 15 minutes.

Serving your Tomato and Herb Seabass
Serve hot atop a bed of fresh spinach leaves.

DASH Diet Friendly Recipes for Weight Loss and Hypertension Recovery

Breakfast

Almond, Blueberry and Cinnamon 'Good Morning' Breakfast Bakes

Ingredients

¼ cup of slivered almonds

1 tablespoon of almond butter

2 cups of gluten-free oats

¼ cup of dried blueberries

4 tablespoons of honey

1 teaspoon of chia seeds

1 ½ teaspoon of baking powder

1 teaspoon of ground cinnamon

½ teaspoon of vanilla extract

2 cups of coconut milk

A small pinch of salt

Method

1. In a bowl, mix together the oats, baking powder, and salt.

2. In a separate large bowl combine the honey, blueberries, chia seeds, cinnamon, coconut milk, vanilla extract and half of the slivered almonds.

3. Add the oats, baking powder and salt to the mix and stir thoroughly.

4. Pre-heat the oven to 370°F.

5. Lightly grease a baking tray with oil.

6. Evenly place the mix into the baking tray. Sprinkle on the remaining slivered almonds.

7. Bake for 25 minutes.

8. Lightly spread the almond butter on top of the bake and place back in the oven for a further 2-4 minutes.

9. Remove to the oven and place in a safe place to
    cool.

**Serving your Almond, Blueberry and Cinnamon
Good Morning Breakfast Bakes**
These breakfast bakes are perfect for those with little
time, cook up a batch and eat this portable breakfast
treat throughout the week.

Smoked Salmon and Runny Egg on Toast

Ingredients
1 pack of smoked salmon
Thick cut gluten-free bread
1 Large egg per person
A small pinch of Salt and ground pepper to taste
1 tablespoon of unsalted butter
Method
2. Heat the butter in a non-stick frying pan or skillet over a medium-high heat.
3. Whilst the butter is melting place the bread under the grill, cook for3-4 minutes (or until toasted) turning midway.
4. Break the eggs and gently slide them into the pan, lower the heat to medium-low and cook until the whites become stiff and the yolk thickens.
5. Remove the salmon from the pack season with a little salt and ground pepper to taste.

Serving your Smoked Salmon and Runny Egg on Toast
Serve immediately, place the salmon on toast and place an egg on top.

Citrus, Almond and Blueberry Salad with Ginger and Greek Yoghurt

Ingredients
1 Valencia orange, peeled and segmented
2 mandarins, peeled and segmented
1 pink grapefruit, peeled and segmented
½ cup of dried cranberries
½ cup of candied/crystallised ginger, crushed
½ cup of blueberries
¼ cup of brown sugar
¼ teaspoon of cinnamon
2 tablespoons of honey
1 ½ cups of natural Greek yoghurt
½ cup of sliced almonds
Method
1. Place the orange, grapefruit and mandarin segments in a bowl cut them into halves (cut the grapefruit segments into thirds) and transfer the cut segments and any juice into a serving bowl.
2. Add the blueberries, cranberries honey and cinnamon, mix well and refrigerate for at least an hour.

Serving your Citrus, Almond and Blueberry Salad with Ginger and Greek Yoghurt
Serve refrigerated with 2 tablespoons of Greek yoghurt.

Buckwheat Granola

Ingredients

1 cup buckwheat

2 cups oats

¼ cup sunflower seeds

¼ cup chia seeds

1 ½ cups pitted dates

5 tablespoons coconut oil

4 ½ tablespoons cacao powder

½ inch piece of ginger, grated

¼ cup apple puree

¼ cup honey

1 teaspoon cinnamon

Method

1. Heat the apple puree, ginger, dates and coconut oil in a saucepan over a medium heat for 5 minutes.

2. In a large bowl mix together the buckwheat, oats, sunflower seeds and chia seeds and put to one side.

3. Remove the date/apple mix from the heat and pour the mix into a blender with the cacao powder until smooth. Pour the smooth mix over the granola, add the honey to the oats and seeds mix and stir well to ensure all the granola mix is coated.

4. Line a baking tray with parchment paper, pour and spread the granola mix evenly in the tray and bake in a pre-heated oven at 350°F180°C

(gas mark 4) for 40-45 minutes turning
regularly.

5. Once lightly toasted remove the granola mix
    from the oven and put to one side to cool, it
    can then be stored for around 3 weeks.

Serving your Buckwheat Granola
Serve with berries and Greek yoghurt or almond milk (4
servings).

Blueberry and Coconut Porridge

Ingredients
1 ½ cups oats
3 cups coconut milk
3 tablespoons cocoa powder
¼ cup blueberries
½ a banana sliced
Honey to taste
2 tablespoons coconut shavings
2 tablespoons of chia seeds
1 tablespoon of slivered almonds

Method
1. Place the oats, chia seeds, coconut milk, cocoa powder into a saucepan and simmer over a medium heat for 5 minutes or until the oats are cooked.
2. Mix in the honey and blueberries and pour into a serving bowl.

Serving your Blueberry and Coconut Porridge
Top the porridge with the banana slices, coconut shavings, slivered almonds and serve hot.

Dinner

Mediterranean Style Tuna Salad

Ingredients
2 tins of tuna in spring water
¼ cup mixed olives
¼ cup finely chopped red onion
¼ cup chopped oven roasted red pepper
3 cherry tomatoes, chopped
150g spinach leaves
1 handful chopped lettuce
A ¼ handful of chopped basil leaves
A pinch of cayenne pepper
1 tablespoon of olive oil
Low-fat mayonnaise (optional)

Method

1. Using a large bowl mix the tuna, lettuce, tomatoes, olives, onion, red pepper, basil, olive oil, and a little cayenne pepper to taste.

2. At this point, it is optional to add 2-3 tablespoons of low-fat mayonnaise.

Serving your Mediterranean Style Tuna Salad
Serve chilled atop a bed of mixed green leaves.

Spicy Carrot and Tomato Soup

Ingredients
2 large tomatoes, chopped
1 packet of sun-dried tomatoes, chopped
2 Large carrots peeled and chopped
1 red chili pepper, chopped
1 large onion, chopped
3 sticks of celery
2 cloves of garlic finely chopped
1 teaspoon of dried cumin
1 tablespoon of tomato puree
1 teaspoon medium heat chili powder
½ teaspoon paprika
Salt and ground black pepper to taste
800ml chicken stock
Olive oil
Method
1. Heat a little olive oil in a saucepan over a medium heat and throw in the onion, garlic and cook for 2 minutes stirring throughout
2. Mix in the chicken stock, tomatoes, carrots, chili pepper, celery, cumin, tomato puree, chili powder, paprika and a little salt and ground black pepper to taste.
3. Simmer for 18 minutes.
4. Blend until smooth using a food processor, return to a low heat and cook for 3-5 minutes.

Serving your Spicy Carrot and Tomato Soup
Serve hot with a gluten-free bread roll.

Thai Steamed Trout

Ingredients
2-4 trout fillets, deboned
2 cloves of garlic, grated
½ inch piece of ginger, grated
¼ teaspoon medium-heat chili flakes
1 ½ teaspoon mixed Thai spice
1 teaspoon lemon juice
½ tablespoon soy sauce
1 tablespoon sesame oil
A pinch of salt and some ground black pepper to taste
Method
1. In a bowl mix together the sesame oil, soy sauce, lemon juice, garlic, ginger, chili flakes, Thai spice and a little salt and pepper to taste.
2. Place the trout in the marinade, ensuring the fillets are fully coated and refrigerate for at least 2 hours.
3. Make a bed from tin foil, place the trout fillets inside and pour over the marinade.
4. Wrap the foil over, covering the trout and place in a pre-heated oven at 400°F/200°C (gas mark 6) for 15-18 minutes.

Serving your Thai Steamed Trout
Serve immediately with brown rice or baked potato and mixed green leaves.

Garlic Chicken and Broccoli Stir-Fry

Ingredients

400g pre-cooked chicken thighs cut into thin slices or cubes

2 cups of broccoli florets

1 cup of green beans, chopped

1 onion, chopped

1 medium-sized carrot, peeled and sliced julienne

1 cup of kale leaves, washed and chopped

2 garlic cloves, finely chopped

1 red pepper, sliced

1 teaspoon of turmeric

½ inch piece of fresh ginger, grated

2 tablespoons of wheat free tamari

1 tablespoon of fresh lemon juice

½ teaspoon of salt

½ teaspoon of ground black pepper

1 tablespoon of apple cider vinegar

1 ½ tablespoons of coconut oil

Method

6. Warm a frying pan over a medium-high heat, toss in and melt the coconut oil.

7. Add the garlic, red pepper, ginger and onion to the pan. Cook for 5-6 minutes.

8. Stir the chicken into the pan and cook for a further 5-6 minutes.

9. Add the turmeric, lemon juice, salt, pepper, carrot, kale leaves, broccoli, green beans and apple cider vinegar to the pan.

10. Stir well and cook over a medium heat for 13-
    15 minutes.

Serving your Garlic Chicken and Broccoli Stir-Fry
Serve with brown rice and a spring onion and green leaf
salad.

Ultimate Salmon Burgers

Ingredients
2 large salmon fillets
2 eggs, beaten
3 clove garlic, grated or minced
1-inch piece ginger, grated or minced
1 teaspoon cumin
½ teaspoon turmeric
¼ cup chopped walnuts
1 tablespoon multi-purpose (gluten-free) flour
1 shallot, finely chopped
Salt and ground black pepper to taste
Olive oil

Method
1. Steam the salmon by wrapping it in tin foil and placing it in a pre-heated oven at 325°F/163°C (gas mark 3) for 8-10 minutes.
2. Remove the salmon from the oven and allow it to cool before placing the fillets into a large mixing bowl and breaking them apart using a fork.
3. Add the eggs, garlic, ginger, cumin, turmeric, walnuts, flour, shallots, and a little salt and pepper to taste to the bowl and mix well.
4. When mixed, use your hands to form the mix into 4-6 burger shapes.

5. Heat 1 tablespoon of olive oil in a frying pan or skillet over a medium heat.

6. Place the salmon burgers into the frying pan and cook for 5-minute turning midway.

Serving your Ultimate Salmon Burgers
Serve with mayonnaise or a squeeze of lemon juice and gluten free bread rolls.

Chicken Noodles and Almond Sauce

Ingredients
400g chicken breast, cubed
¼ cup sliced almonds
1 packet soba noodles
¼ cup almond butter
2 tablespoons honey
1 tablespoons soy sauce
2 tablespoons rice wine vinegar
¼ cup red bell pepper, chopped
¼ cup yellow bell pepper
½ cup spring onions
2 radishes, sliced
Freshwater
A pinch of salt and ground black pepper to taste
Olive oil
Method
1. In a bowl whisk together the vinegar, honey, almond butter and soy sauce.
2. Season the chicken with some salt and pepper. Heat some olive oil in a large frying pan, toss in the chicken and cook for 8 minutes. Drain away any excess water or fats.
3. Add the spring onions, peppers and radishes and cook for a further 8 minutes, tossing throughout.

4. Whilst the chicken and vegetables cook, cook
    the noodles as per the instructions on the
    packet.
5. Drain the noodles, place in a bowl alongside the
    chicken and vegetable mix.

Serving your Chicken Noodles and Almond Sauce
Stir well and serve with a sprinkling of sliced almonds.

Indian Style Chicken and Potato Curry

400g chicken, cubed
350g Maris Piper or Russet potatoes peeled and roughly cut into quarters
1 white onion chopped
3 cloves of garlic finely chopped
1 ½ inch piece of ginger, grated
1 ½ teaspoon garam masala
1 tin of chopped tomatoes
½ teaspoon medium heat chili powder
½ teaspoon cumin
¼ teaspoon coriander
½ teaspoon turmeric
1 tablespoon of olive oil
Salt and ground black pepper to taste
¼ cup of water

Method

1. Heat the olive oil in a large saucepan over a medium-high heat, when hot, throw in the onions, garlic, ginger and cook on a medium heat for 1-2 minutes.

2. Add chicken, garam masala, chili powder, cumin, coriander, turmeric and salt and pepper to taste and stir well.

3. Pour the tin of chopped tomatoes and water and add the potatoes into to saucepan, stir well.

4. Cook on a medium heat for 30-35 minutes or until the cooking liquids have reduced by half.

Serving your Indian Style Chicken and Potato Curry

Serve hot with rice and gluten-free chapatti/roti

Lemon and Herb Cod Loin

Ingredients
2-4 cod loin fillets
1 small handful of chopped basil leaves
1 ½ teaspoons of Italian mixed herbs
¼ cup chopped parsley
1 tablespoon of lemon juice
1 tablespoon of lime juice
2 tablespoons of olive oil
Salt and ground black pepper to taste
Method
1. Mix together the basil, Italian mixed herbs, lemon juice, lime juice, chopped parsley, olive oil and a little salt and pepper to taste.
2. Coat the cod loins in the mix, cover and refrigerate for at least 30 minutes.
3. Heat some olive oil in a pan over a medium heat.
4. Place the cod loins into the pan, pour over any remaining marinade and cook for 4-6 minutes, turning midway.

Serving Lemon and Herb Cod Loin
Serve with rice, spoon the juices from the pan over the cod and rice.

Vegetarian and Vegan Recipes

One Pot Quinoa and Broccoli

Ingredients
3 cups broccoli florets
1 cup quinoa
1 onion, finely chopped
3 cloves of garlic, grated
1 shallot, finely chopped
800ml vegetable stock
1 tablespoon balsamic vinegar
2 teaspoons Italian mixed herbs
Salt and ground black pepper to taste
1 tablespoon olive oil
1 cup grated cheese of choice (optional)
Method

4. Heat some olive oil in a saucepan over a medium heat. Throw the onions, garlic, shallot, balsamic vinegar and Italian mixed herbs into the saucepan and cook for 3 minutes.

5. Add the quinoa to the saucepan along with a little salt and ground black pepper to taste, cook for 1-2 minutes before pouring the vegetable stock into the saucepan, cover and cook for 10 minutes.

6. Add the broccoli to the pan, replace the cover and cook over a low heat for a further 8-10 minutes.

Serving your One Pot Quinoa and Broccoli
Stir in the grated cheese (optional) and serve immediately.

Citrus, Avocado and Green Leaf Salad

Ingredients

½ pink grapefruit peeled, sliced and segmented

1 Valencia orange peeled, sliced and segmented

1 tablespoon of finely grated or minced shallots

1 avocado, sliced

Mixed fresh salad greens

1 handful of spinach leaves

½ teaspoon of Dijon mustard

2 tablespoons of red wine vinegar

2 tablespoons olive oil

¼ cup sliced almonds

A small pinch of salt and ground black pepper to taste

Method

1. In a bowl, whisk together the Dijon mustard, olive oil, shallots and red wine vinegar with a little salt and ground black pepper to taste.

2. Mix the pink grapefruit, oranges, avocado, spinach and green leaves in a bowl.

Serving your Citrus, Avocado and Green Leaf Salad

Toss the vinaigrette with the salad and serve.

Classic Veggie Burgers

Ingredients
1 large sweet potato
½ cup red onion, finely chopped
2 cloves of garlic, grated
1/2 cup quinoa
¼ cup multi-purpose gluten-free flour
½ cup black beans
¼ cup kidney beans
½ teaspoon cumin
¼ teaspoon paprika
2 teaspoons Cajun spice
Olive oil
½ cup watercress
1 cup lettuce
A pinch of salt and ground black pepper to taste
Method
1. Cook the quinoa as per the instructions on the pack.
2. Roast the sweet potato for 30 minutes (or until soft) in a pre-heated oven at 400°F/200°C (gas mark 6).
3. Allow the sweet potato to cool, remove the skin, place in a food processor alongside the garlic, red onions, paprika, Cajun spice, cumin, kidney beans, black beans and salt and pepper to taste. Blend until almost smooth.
4. In a large bowl, mix together the sweet potato mix and quinoa along with a little flour (just enough so that burger shapes can be formed.

5. Divide the mix into 6-8 burger or patty shapes
    and refrigerate for 30 minutes.

6. Heat some olive oil in a frying pan or skillet and
    cook the burger for 5-6 minutes on either side
    or until they begin to brown.

Serving your Classic Veggie Burgers
Serve topped with lettuce and cress inside gluten free
burger buns.

Seasonal Root Vegetable Tagine

Ingredients
400ml vegetable stock
1 bunch of carrots, roughly chopped
1 cup of kale
2 sweet potatoes, roughly chopped
2 parsnips, roughly chopped
1 large leek, roughly chopped
1 large red onion, chopped
½ teaspoon coriander
½ teaspoon cumin
½ teaspoon cinnamon
¼ teaspoon cayenne pepper
2 cloves of garlic, finely chopped
1-inch piece of ginger, grated or minced
2 tablespoons tomato puree
1 tablespoon lemon juice
Salt and ground black pepper
Olive oil
¼ cup chopped almonds

Method

1. Heat some olive oil in a large saucepan over a medium heat and cook the chopped onions for 2 minutes.

2. Add the parsnips to the saucepan and cook for 3 minutes before tossing in the almonds, cumin, coriander, cinnamon, cayenne, garlic, ginger, tomato puree and a little salt and pepper to taste.

3. Pour the vegetable stock into the pan along
    with the rest of the vegetables, bring to the boil
    and simmer for 18 minutes or until vegetables
    begin to soften.

Serving your Seasonal Root Vegetable Tagine
Serve garnished with chopped almonds and bulgur
wheat or quinoa.

Chilli Pumpkin Soup

Ingredients

3 cups of butternut squash, chopped
2 large russet or Maris Piper potato, peeled and chopped
1 onion, chopped
2 celery sticks, chopped
3 cloves of garlic, finely chopped
1-inch piece of ginger, grated
2 red chilies, chopped
1 teaspoon of garam masala
¼ teaspoon cumin
¼ teaspoon coriander
¼ teaspoon ground black pepper
Salt to taste
800ml chicken stock
1 tablespoon of olive oil

Method

1. In a large cooking pot, warm the olive oil over a medium heat. Add the onions, garlic, cumin, coriander, ground black pepper, chilies and ginger and cook for 2 minutes.
2. Add the butternut squash, celery, potato and a little salt to taste and the chicken stock, stir well.
3. Bring to the boil, lower the heat and simmer for 10 minutes.
4. Lower the heat and cook for a further 15-18 minutes.
5. Using a submersion blender or food processor, blend the soup until smooth.

Serving your Chili Pumpkin Soup
Serve hot (serves 4).

Free Bonus Book

Evie has written a number of healthy cookbooks and recipe guides and now receiving your FREE book couldn't be easier. For your FREE printable pdf book simply send an email to
sadisticallydeliciousseries@gmail.com